Surviving the
ICU

A Tool Kit for the Critical Care Nurse

RACHEL LARCOM,

MSN, FNP-BC, CCRN

ISBN 979-8-88644-598-5 (Paperback)
ISBN 979-8-88644-599-2 (Digital)

Covenant Books
11661 Hwy 707
Murrells Inlet, SC 29576
www.covenantbooks.com

Contents

Introduction

Surviving the ICU

As you walk into your new job with great anticipation, you envision all the experiences you might encounter as an ICU nurse. Whether for the higher complexity of patient situations or just a desire to challenge yourself and expand your experience, your aspirations are most likely high. Amidst the excitement of learning new things and accomplishing your initial goals, there may be occasional frustrations that arise from self-doubt and disappointment. Even if your experience is mostly positive, these feelings are normal and part of the growing process. Receiving the new knowledge required for the critical care setting combined with its application to patient care and responsibilities can be overwhelming.

These challenges range from acclimating to a new team and unit routine with advanced patient care to managing conflict with patients, families, team members, and even providers. The fact is that the expectations of the ICU nurse are higher, patient conditions could change at any moment, and you have to be ready to act on evolving situations. At any level of experience, there will be some degree of challenge and conflict. Over time, learning the management of conflict gives way to identifying which battles are worth fighting for and where to exercise flexibility. Most of the time, all it takes is remembering commonsense principles; however, entering into intense situations can make one easily forget even the simplest of common knowledge.

Even for those boasting excellent adaptability, the ICU environment can serve as an incredible source of stress for many reasons. Studies have proven that nurse burnout has a high prevalence in the ICU setting, contributing to nurses leaving the profession as well as safety concerns in patient care, toxic work environments, and so forth. Similarly, research has shown that there are incredible, effective solutions for preventing and combating burnout. The survival skills included in this text will provide you with the tools necessary to do so by understanding conflict management, learning emotional intelligence, and managing stress with practical tips to survive *and* thrive in this environment. Similar to when training in the wilderness or preparing for battle, working in the ICU requires strategy and awareness of your surroundings.

Adapted from military and wilderness survival tactics with additional nursing applications, I have found these skills to be vital for success when entering the critical care environment, as some shifts feel like active battle and others as if you are out in the wilderness. This is not an exhaustive list, but it will augment other resources you gain along the way. You have answered the call, stepped up to the plate, and advanced into the hardest role you will ever love. As you take hold of these skills, know that you have what it takes to succeed. And most of all, know that you bring something unique, valuable, and necessary to the team. I encourage you to take the time to evaluate these skills, even if you feel they may not be necessary. Whatever the amount of time you ultimately serve as a critical care nurse, let these principles be a valuable piece of your experience and nursing journey.

How to Survive

8 Tactics to Succeed and Thrive in the ICU Setting

1

Know Your Cover and When to Take Cover

Knowing your cover and when to take cover are foundational to working in any environment. For example, in the military, a soldier must be aware of who in their unit is covering them as it could be a matter of life or death. Each one is trained to understand the protocols and strategies to use so they can maneuver in any situation that arises. Similarly, prior to preparing for time in the wilderness, one must have an understanding of the landscape, how to call for help, what to do in the case of injury, and so forth. One has to take cover during inclement weather in the wilderness and during active attack in battle. This usually involves finding shelter, camouflaging in the setting, and the like. In every health-care system, there are policies, procedures, and clinical standards that create a framework for patient care as derived from evidence-based practice.

These are also in place as a safeguard, or covering, for the nurse in case of and for the prevention of errors, near misses, and other events. While the intensity is not to the same degree as that of a soldier, knowing these processes is especially key to success for nurses in the ICU setting. This may be a simple reminder; however, it is a vital tactic for remaining up-to-date on the latest guidelines and, ultimately, ensuring the safest care for your patients. Your preceptor(s) and those in leadership will guide you to the policies and procedures to focus on when researching for your unit via your facility database. These serve as backup and protection, keeping team members accountable for what is included in safe and consistent patient care.

Taking cover includes using the protections set in place and submitting to those in authority. This involves knowing the proper chain of command, which is vital for accountability and taking the appropriate steps for process improvement. In the case where patient safety is a concern when following established standards and protocols, therein lies the responsibility to reassess the process for improvement. This involves voicing concerns to those at the level above you and working together for effective solutions. At times, you may need to take additional steps toward those further up the chain of command. If this is the case, as you approach those involved, ensure your argument and/or suggestions are supported by evidence-based practice or at least have trusted resources to back you up. This may include taking time to research current evidence and standards.

When acting in these situations, the main priority is patient safety with consideration of scope of practice and nurse safety. Becoming familiar with your state's Nurse Practice Act is also helpful in knowing your cover, and when in doubt, consult with your leadership. We need to be aware of what is within our scope and outside our scope, not just for litigation's sake but really for the safety of the patient. Mainly, it matters that we know what we are doing. These principles apply to knowing the routine processes to follow and for when you are concerned regarding safety and outdated practice.

2

Win the 15-Second Fight

The Only Easy Day Was Yesterday

There is a tactic from the military to win the fifteen-second fight, where the first fifteen seconds of the overall battle are the most crucial. This is where battle strategy is established and the plans are set into motion. Because the battle ensues and time cannot be wasted, these fifteen seconds will require focus and determination. Regarding the ICU, this is the time frame just after huddle (if applicable) and during and immediately following report. There are multiple factors that impact the attitude of the day and could threaten defeat, making this a crucial fight to win.

In this process, the nurse is gathering the data necessary to strategize for the fight of the day. The goal is to win the day and not let the day win within reasonable expectations. As all nurses know too well, anything can happen during the shift, especially in the ICU. Therefore, this is the time to prepare and strategize for the constants in the shift, such as:

- ❖ Knowing who is assigned around you for break coverage and assistance;
- ❖ Active orders, tasks, and medications to develop priority list;
- ❖ Required level of monitoring for patient assignment;
- ❖ Providers available / on call;
- ❖ Having items ready of what to report to provider;
- ❖ Acknowledging the status of the unit and if others have heavy loads; and
- ❖ Taking a deep breath and knowing who you can call for help.

These items will establish your plan to prepare you for the changes that come throughout the shift. While the process will obviously exceed fifteen seconds, the principle remains and makes space for staying alert to what is going on around you. As a result, you are adaptable and have a realistic view of where you can lend a hand in helping the team. There will be shifts where your assignment will limit you from being available to assist other nurses. However, maintaining your load will keep the unit moving smoothly, and it will keep you from overextending yourself while still being a team player.

This crucial step of the shift will set you up for success in flexibility, being open to growth with continued learning, and staying alert to respond effectively. Sometimes you have to embrace the suck (as the military says), making the best of what you have been given in a stressful, challenging, and variable environment. There are times when the day wins and the inevitable occurs during your shift that you did not expect with results you could not control. As long as you give your best and you give your all, you have nothing to be ashamed of. For that is when you have truly won the fifteen-second fight.

3

Conflict Management

Understanding effective conflict management is one of the most critical tools to surviving the ICU. Conflict is a part of life, providing the opportunity for growth and change or potentially furthering frustration and burnout. The way conflict is handled and approached will determine the result. A point to consider is found in the acronym HALT, which is used to describe the factors that make one vulnerable to the negative effects of conflict: hungry, angry, lonely, tired. Being cognizant of these vulnerabilities and making the effort to prevent negative consequences when experiencing them is a vital start to approaching conflict in a healthy way.

Within a team, conflict can bring members together as problems are worked out or create division from festering frustration, potentially leading to toxic work environments. There are many contributing factors to conflict for various reasons and motivations. Taking a moment to understand the potential consequences of conflict management is crucial in effectively preventing burnout and surviving the challenges of the ICU environment.

When experiencing difficult situations amidst the ICU team, disrespect and harassment should not be tolerated. However, for various reasons, negative behavior between nurses and other team members can be assumed as "the normal" or just accepted over time, rather than actively prevented and dealt with. There are effective and useful tools available to prevent incivility in the workplace. Your facility should have zero tolerance protocols in place to identify and report harassment, incivility, and bullying that will ultimately create healthy work environments when followed. These also apply to patient behavior toward staff members.

If you cannot find the protocols, there are great resources found on the American Association of Critical Care Nurses website that can be implemented. Encountering and managing these situations may not be a challenge for some; however, for many nurses in the ICU setting, conflict from harassment, incivility, disagreements, and so forth is incredibly difficult. When there is no resolve, each situation can build upon the previous and ultimately lead to early burnout, contributing to increased job turnover rates and self-harm behaviors in some cases. Simply acknowledging that conflict exists and arming yourself with emotional intelligence is the start to succeeding in this area.

Speaking up in a respectful manner when you know something is wrong is an important tactic as you are your best advocate. Respect opens the door to being respected, and respecting yourself helps your confidence to grow. As you stand up for yourself and set boundaries when interacting with others, you will see which battles are worth the energy and which ones to just let go. With experience, this becomes clearer, and support from those who have been through similar circumstances is also helpful. It is good to acknowledge your frustrations in an effort to come to terms with where you stand and how you feel, and then express yourself in a healthy manner and in a safe place.

Journaling is an excellent tool for expressing your thoughts without unnecessarily off-loading to someone who does not understand and/or may use it against you. Or you may like to use an outlet such as art, music, and the like. A good rule of thumb to know if something is worth reporting is to do so when patient safety is of concern, you have been attacked, and/or your boundaries have been violated. If communicating with that person does not lead to an effective resolution, then it is time to take the issue up the chain of command. It may not seem worth the fight at times, but if you find yourself anxious and unable to move on from the situation, it would be worth at least a conversation with your manager.

> *What areas of conflict have you encountered*
> *so far in your nursing career?*
> *What outlets of expression or hobbies have you used*
> *to work through conflict and challenging situations?*

Conflict also arises within patient situations and with family members. For example, your patient load may be heavy, and patients and/or family members do not understand the dynamics of the balance of patient care in your assignment. You will often be communicating with them over the telephone, which adds to their questions and frustrations because they cannot be with the patient in person. Most of the time, it is due to not being exposed to the hospital setting and/or emotional responses to not being in control of what is going on with their loved one. In reality, unless an individual has firsthand experience working in the bedside environment, they will have difficulty seeing the full picture and knowing where we are coming from.

Unfortunately, their expectations of how care is or should be completed will differ from what is truly encompassed in your role as the bedside nurse in the ICU. Families and even patients will not always understand the process of notifying providers, addressing critical situations, following specific protocols, and so on, and they may react out of misunderstanding. They will often project their anxiety on nurses and ask with urgency for something that is not high on the priority list for the patient, such as water or a blanket and the like. This is where conflict may occur as they become agitated. It can be difficult as the primary nurse to remain calm while being firm in communicating priorities and explaining rationales to the patient and/or family.

There are times when it will not be worth the continual attempt to rationalize as you speak to a proverbial brick wall. At these moments, take a deep breath and do your best to be professional and say only what you need to for the conversation. They do not need to completely understand our full process and may not understand the complexity of the clinical situation as there are multiple factors involved. I have found that when you begin the conversation by setting boundaries with a pleasant but firm approach, the anxiety mostly subsides enough to establish a rapport with even those who are very upset.

Be confident with what you are explaining, and it may require taking the time to remind them that you are there to take care of the patient. Sometimes being up front with that statement will remind them that their loved one is in good hands. It is also good to keep in mind that we cannot win over everyone, but it is still important to do our best to explain the situation and keep the patient first. Other confrontations with patients and families may occur; however, these are the most common.

While it may not always be conflict-related, when the shift presents one thing seemingly after another, I cannot stress enough the importance of leaning on the support of your team members. Some days will come when you will feel alone, and even those around you are just as busy. It can be difficult to not take it personally; however, especially in these moments, reach out to your charge nurse and/or other resource members with clear communication of what you need help with. The circumstances of the ICU setting are often chaotic, with multiple critical situations occurring at the same time.

Assigning patients and addressing concerns throughout the shift requires a level of multitasking from the charge nurse and others. Therefore, it is important to not be quick to judge in thinking you are being ignored or assume what else may be going on. That is why I emphasize reaching out for help when needed and being helpful as well. I have found that in the moments I assumed people did not want to help or I was not being checked on, once I asked for help or checked on those nurses, there was something else going on that I did not realize. That helped me understand the situation.

There are occasions when individuals are not proactive in helping; however, if you continue to seek help or find ways to help them, they will eventually come around. Once again, we cannot win everyone over and "fix" everyone, but we can be *our* best and impart to those around us the goodness of helping others. We are on a continual journey of learning and improving as individuals *and* as nurses. We should always remain open to those opportunities to shine and inspire however they present in our lives.

Remember that you are a part of the team, and there is a purpose for you being with your patient assignment beyond just being picked or placed with them for that shift. You have what it takes to succeed and care for your patients as well as help your team. As you reflect on this truth, you can effectively manage conflict and make the right decisions that help you grow stronger and more adaptable within the ICU environment. This also helps when dealing with leaders and preceptors throughout your orientation period and into your career.

There will be times when what is asked of you will vary from the previous preceptor or leader because of their flow or routine, and this can be a source of frustration for you. Instead, let it be a learning opportunity for you. As long as what is being asked of you is not against the standard of care and does not threaten patient safety, do your best to breathe through the frustration and complete the task. Though the variances may seem to be conflicting or you feel you are being corrected, you should be able to speak with them openly and discuss any necessary clarification. Sometimes just asking the right questions respectfully allows for further open communication and a better working team because of mutual understanding.

Moving past the initial reaction will sometimes help you to see where you may want to adjust your routine or where you need to see the patient situation from a different perspective. You may have heard the phrase "Eat the chicken and leave the bone." This relates to circumstances of conflict (and to life in general) as you do your best to take from a difficult situation that which is good for you and leave the things that hinder your growth and momentum toward your goals. The worst thing you can do is to let it fester and turn into bitterness or a source of gossip.

Choose to see the good, and if there seems to be none, do your best to remain professional and respectful. We are responsible for our own outlook, growth, perspective, and change. When it seems someone else is making you frustrated or feel like your outlook is changing to something negative, take a moment to evaluate why and see if it only requires a shift in perspective. It will not always be easy or a quick change; however, it will be worth it to live your best life.

Have you experienced any situations where preceptors varied in instruction and you became frustrated? If so, what made you most frustrated and why? What is a positive you can take from the experience?

The positive and negative effects of conflict are dependent upon the perspective and attitude used when approached by it. For example, conflict can be positive in improving working relationships as long as there is open communication and mutual respect among team members. This occurs when boundaries are established, rules are well-known and followed, and members choose to find the best in one another with encouragement and process improvement. Unfortunately, the opposite is miscommunication, damaged relationships, and a distrusting climate, which is often precipitated by gossip and slander.

While many other individuals choose these negative behaviors to gain status or for other reasons, you do not have to respond or feel pressured to choose to use them against someone else. It is difficult to walk away from them at times, especially when feeling defensive and you see how it is affecting relationships. However, it is possible and healthy to set boundaries as they occur, redirecting your focus to the important things, such as patient care and promoting a healthy work environment. It may seem like contributing to the gossip is the right and/or natural solution in the moment, especially when you feel it is the only way to get along in the unit.

However, gossip and slander are destructive, and you cannot expect to not be talked about if you continue to engage in the practice yourself. Rather, it will continue a trend of negativity if allowed to continue. Instead, choose to do what you know is right and allow these situations to strengthen you rather than bring you down. Think of good qualities in others and encourage them in those areas. In doing so, you will continue sowing seeds of positivity that will eventually contribute to improved working environments. When it feels as though there are only a small number of nurses, if any, whom you can be open with, focus on those you know you can positively impact and upon your patients, those who you know appreciate your care. Your energy is then geared toward improving your environment and turning challenging situations into positive growth and change.

What is another situation of conflict you have experienced that comes to mind right now? As you reflect upon that situation, what positive experience can you see as a result (i.e., growth, change in dynamics of workflow, opportunities for learning, etc.)?

4

Survive and Thrive in Any Environment

Identifying Burnout and Its Warning Signs

Burnout is defined by *Webster's Dictionary* as "exhaustion of physical or emotional strength or motivation, usually as a result of prolonged stress or frustration"[1] (*Merriam-Webster Inc.*, 2020). There are multiple contributing factors to burnout, especially in the ICU setting, thereby creating multiple strategies to

---

[1] Merriam-Webster. (n.d.). Burnout. In *Merriam-Webster.com dictionary*. Retrieved April 1, 2021, from https://www.merriam-webster.com/dictionary/burnout.

prevent and combat it. In the military, if a soldier is experiencing burnout, it could compromise their ability to effectively complete the mission, perform their duties, and so forth. The same is true for nurses in the ICU setting.

From the moment the report is given, the shift is often busy, and you hit the ground running. There are multiple demands for your attention and many factors to consider in the matter of one shift, in addition to just caring for yourself. Taking the time to understand burnout and its lasting effects will improve your outlook as an ICU nurse and allow you to make the most of your time and experience. Preventing burnout has been proven to increase staff retention and improve conflict management, among other positive effects. In this section, we will consider the tactics necessary to identify, prevent, and combat burnout, as well as its warning signs.

The warning signs of burnout often occur subtly and could easily be overlooked for a long time if not recognized and dealt with early on. One of the signs includes instances when the expectations or ideals of the employee differ from the reality of the position, eventually leading to the loss of their ability to adapt to their environment. For instance, this could be as simple as becoming familiar with new tasks or learning the dynamics of the physician-nurse relationship within the ICU. Whether due to intimidation, arrogance, or simply the frustrations of learning the new flow, unfulfilled expectations could be a challenging obstacle contributing to early burnout and a delay in personal and professional growth.

Other potential causes of burnout include moral distress and compassion fatigue. Moral distress occurs for different reasons, such as when the nurse knows the right and ethical decision to make for their patient but feels they cannot move in that direction. Two of the most common examples include when family or a physician continues care for a patient with a poor prognosis or when a patient's wishes are not being honored. These tend to cause the most stress for nurses in the ICU as we feel powerless to honor our patients in their care. Other risks to moral distress include self-doubt, anxiety related to conflict, external pressures, and/or power imbalances.

Additionally, compassion fatigue may cause burnout resulting from compassion being reduced over time and a constant desire to help those who are suffering, especially when there is perceived delivery of inappropriate care. While the situations leading up to these risks vary, the sequelae can be the same. Desiring to help others and being a part of someone's journey in their critically ill state is not only natural, it is honorable. All the aspects of the essence of nursing are valuable. However, if there is not an avenue of resting our minds and an outlet to release tension, the emotions that accompany the experience of caring for others in critical and intense situations can lead to exhaustion that will take time to recover from.

Furthermore, it is okay to be human and that we give ourselves the grace to not only make mistakes but also be affected by the world around us. We need to be strong, but it should not be at the cost of losing ourselves in the process. It is vital that we are involved and voice our concerns about patient care and being emotionally involved within safe and professional boundaries. The risk of burnout is present when it is repetitively difficult to find the balance of knowing when to step into and when to step back from a situation. This understanding improves with time, experience, and leaning on the support of those who have been through similar situations before.

So how do we recognize the warning signs of burnout? Burnout affects individuals psychologically and physically and should raise red flags in the case of a consistent occurrence. In a fast-paced, high-stress environment, it is understandable to be fatigued and overwhelmed on occasion in relation to the workload. However, when these symptoms begin to increase on a more consistent basis, it is time to look further for other warning signs. For example, anxiety, frustration, and feeling overwhelmed are common, especially when beginning in the ICU. These will typically subside as nurses become more familiar with the routine, lean on others for support, and gain a greater understanding of what is required of them.

When these symptoms lead to unprofessional behavior, the inability to feel happy, having a lack of empathy, and feeling inadequate at work, then it is time to take a step back and come to terms with what the workload has been and how the experience has affected perspective and mindset. The same goes for physical symptoms that go beyond the occasional fatigue, soreness, and tension that occur after a busy or rough day. It becomes worrisome when they lead to insomnia, consistent muscle tension, headaches, gastrointestinal problems, and other physical ailments that do not easily resolve.

As you review these symptoms, do any stick out to you that you have experienced as a nurse?

The same tactics used for preventing burnout are also used to combat it. There are many things we come across as nurses in the ICU setting that are beyond our control (such as management decisions, patient outcomes, and others' behaviors), yet they affect us over time if we let them. The factors that we can control, however, include how we handle the stressors and challenges we face, how we prepare ourselves for the battlefield, and how we recover to process what we have experienced in the fight, so to speak. Preventing and combating burnout begins with taking care of ourselves. This is a simple concept that is not always easy to complete.

As nurses, the effort to take care of others can often take precedence over our own needs and getting our rest. This is where it is necessary to find the work-life balance for our own quality of life. A simple measure you could do to start this process includes making a list of what needs to be done for the week, tasks to complete for days off, and so forth. Having hobbies, socializing with friends and family, and intentionally making other time for relaxation are important strategies for taking your mind off work and unwinding enough so you can continue facing the day in the ICU. This also includes utilizing paid time off and limiting the number of days worked consecutively, especially when just beginning on the unit.

Finding the right rhythm and flow of your schedule and making the effort to take time off when needed is key in preventing yourself from getting overwhelmed and overburdened with work. We need to have that time away and separate from the work routine so we can recalibrate and gain a healthy perspective. Through my time in the ICU, I was strategic about when and if I should pick up overtime because I knew to recognize when it would be too much. We all know the struggles of dealing with a short-staffed shift. However, we would not be good for anybody if we worked so hard and had nothing left to give. If you are one that would be able to pick up extra shifts, just keep that in mind so that you do not stretch yourself too thin and contribute to potential burnout.

There are resources available, such as cognitive therapy, meditation techniques, and support groups, if needed, for assistance in coping with stress and taking care of ourselves. Other strategies of self-care to consider include time management during work days and when completing the home routine, formal training for stress reduction and assertiveness if needed, and ensuring adequate rest, healthy eating habits, and getting exercise. In the unit, promoting a healthy work environment is also helpful, though challenging when others may not share the same values or positive attitude. However, as you make the effort to improve your work environment, you can know you are doing your part in making it an enjoyable experience and that you will impart positivity to those around you.

We cannot control how others will respond or choose to live their lives. However, we can control our own lives in how we respond and our attitude toward the situation. It is up to us to leave at the door the issues of home so we can focus on work and leave at work the issues of work so we can live a quality life at home. Strategies for preventing and combatting burnout at a unit level include setting realistic and measurable goals for the ICU patients, including the family and close contacts whom the patient chooses, and involving ethics and palliative care when needed for complex situations.

Knowing your resources that are available for your patients is crucial in taking the burden off your shoulders and establishing the appropriate care plan that can be accomplished while honoring their wishes. These are the common issues in the ICU that often lead to overburdening nurses and creating a stressful environment due to the ethical dilemmas and other situations previously mentioned. Our adaptation to the ICU routine, while honoring the wishes of the patient, is an art because of the creative process that takes place to do the right thing for ourselves and the patient.

Nurses have the unique ability to combine the understanding the science of what we do with the compassion of seeing the patients with care to meet all of their needs. As nurses, we see the full picture: from the basic needs and concerns of the patient to the complex pathophysiology of their condition. While our care may not produce the exact results we hope for, reaching out to the appropriate resources and making the effort to complete what we know is right is enough. In utilizing these strategies to combat and prevent burnout, we are positioned to survive and thrive in the ICU as we learn to take care of ourselves in the process of taking care of others.

Do you find it difficult to take care of yourself and ensure mental and emotional health, along with meeting physical needs, while working? Do you feel as though you can apply these strategies mentioned? What other methods have you found helpful in preventing and combating burnout?

5

Increase Survivability

Increasing survivability equips you to be ready for the long haul by arming yourself with the following practical tactics. These will save you from overextending yourself and feeling defeated or out of control because you will be prepared for whatever comes your way *and* be able to enjoy your day! Tackling your practical skills also helps you to appreciate your job and catch the vision of where you are meant to be. These skills include open communication, proactivity and clustering of care, having layers for temperature changes, and other tools for staying nourished and hydrated.

Open communication and appropriate delegation are vital to the health of any team. If in the midst of battle, soldiers do not communicate, fatal mistakes could happen. In the ICU, nurses need to openly communicate and appropriately delegate when in need of help so they and their patients are safe. I know from experience that it can be difficult to ask for help, knowing others have many tasks to do and feeling pressured to get everything done independently because it is your assignment. This is especially true when getting familiar with the routine and remembering all the tasks and orders to complete. It can also be difficult to delegate due to the desire to control the situation at hand. At the end of the day, however, it is not worth the exhaustion and potential burnout if we can help it when there is an opportunity for assistance.

Communicate with your charge nurse if needed and utilize whomever may be available for those tasks to be completed so the patients are taken care of. You are taking care of yourself because you are saving your back from injury, you are free to document so you can leave on time, and you prevent yourself from getting overwhelmed. Realistically, these things do happen; some days you leave late or you feel overwhelmed, but the tactic to remember here is to prevent them from recurring so much that you get burned-out. As a team, nurses work hard *together*, which allows for a cohesive running team because they understand each other. We cannot control every situation; however, leaning upon those who support us will help us adapt, learn from the struggle, and grow into a stronger person.

Time management is another vital tactic that increases survivability. While its mastery is a progressive process, an imperative step is to be proactive in care to save time. This is a reachable goal that can be accomplished at the beginning of your ICU journey. You may have heard it termed clustering care. This involves simply planning the day, as we saw in the fifteen-second fight, and anticipating care as the shift progresses. Of course, with experience, this gets easier. However, you have been given enough information to be off to a good start. A helpful first step is to survey the patient's room each time you enter, taking note of supplies needing replenished, what needs to be organized and exchanged, and what the patient needs, such as water, to obtain upon returning.

This is also connected to prioritizing, which goes hand in hand with time management. Setting your priorities is a constant variable during the shift, as patient acuity may change so frequently amidst the frequent monitoring, vital signs, and other responsibilities that are a part of ICU care. For example, if you have just entered your patient's room to replace a drip bag and your patient is asking for tissues, water, and the TV channel changed, that can wait for you to complete your task. You are not ignoring your patient, but you are addressing the more urgent need among necessary and ongoing tasks. In this case, it would be proactive to ask if they needed anything else and verify if anything else needed changed, such as suction, etc., before leaving the room.

There are many other examples, but I believe you get the point. The main concept to remember is that there will be multiple demands for your attention and response; however, you can successfully answer them as you prioritize effectively. In orientation, you will have your preceptor(s) and others thereafter to refer to for assistance if needed. Be assured that this improves with time, and all it takes is one step forward to get you going. It starts with taking a breath and utilizing your resources to know what tasks and so forth are vital for your focus in that moment.

There are a few other practical tactics that are essential to increasing your survivability that maintain your environment and keep you nourished and flowing throughout the day. For instance, prepare yourself with adequate layers that can be adapted to the temperature you encounter as the shift progresses. As on the battlefield and in the wilderness, one must wear the appropriate clothing and have the spare attire to face the applicable elements. We all know the impact of busy shifts that increase body temperature and the ability for the thermostat to be adjusted, making for a frustrating battle of who is hot and who is cold. In order to survive and operate at your most optimal, bring a jacket you could easily remove, or if you know you will be cold, bring a long sleeve shirt to wear under your uniform top.

Additionally, for those with long hair, bring a hair tie or other useful tool to keep your hair back if you are overheated and when you need to keep it safely out of patient care. While you may be one to tolerate having your hair down while working, it is wise to be prepared for those moments that quickly change the environment. It is better to be prepared in advance for the expected, which then positions one to respond quickly when the unexpected occurs without losing ground or sight of the mission at hand. The focus to remember here is safety and efficiency. Can you accomplish tasks when you're feeling hungry, angry, lazy, and tired *(HALT)*? Most likely, that would be challenging, which leads to the next tactic of hydration and nourishment.

A simple way to ensure you are nourished throughout your shift is to keep snacks that will fit in your pocket. These may include nuts, dried fruit, seeds, protein bars, pretzels, etc. Due to your assignment, you may not have the opportunity to take fifteen-minute breaks or even an adequate lunch break at times. Rather than allowing hunger to cloud your day, keep something with you that you can easily take in as you go. Additionally, keep your water in a place you can get to while still being near your patient assignment. We all know the importance of being well hydrated and nourished; however, we also know the struggle of keeping our patients as cared for as they need. All we can do is give it our best and be as prepared as possible.

6

Train to Survive

Training to survive includes an ongoing process of evaluation of where you stand, how you are doing, and where improvements are needed. This begins with a self-assessment as you begin on the unit, again as you finish orientation and periodically throughout your ICU career. This benefits you and your team because you have a realistic view of your own perspective of where you stand in the team. Your expertise and experience are valuable and necessary to the unit. Taking a self-assessment helps to shift that focus, if needed, so that you are reminded that your role matters. Additionally, you can see the positive impact of the present challenges that will lead to learning opportunities and continual growth.

There are many factors that make this easier said than done. However, this step is vital for you to be the best you can be. Even if the ICU is a stepping stone for you, how you adapt and grow determines your survivability for your nursing career. It is in these challenging times that you gain the skills and perspective of what it takes to be the best version of yourself and do what you have been born to do. Once you can see where you stand, your growth will strengthen and encourage you to encourage others. Sometimes frustration can be productive toward positive, necessary change. However, a negative attitude from frustration, or whatever the case may be, often festers and builds toward burnout if not dealt with.

Many times, our frustrations are warranted, but it is important that we take care of ourselves in regards to mental health and joy. It has been proven that joy and positivity in consistent doses results in more efficiency, healthier minds, and stronger teams. It is not an easy fix, but it is a simple process that starts with bringing joy to your environment and attempting to see the positive in the situation. This is not dismissing what needs to change, nor overlooking wrongdoing, but rather taking a moment to think clearly, objectively, and in a healthy way that promotes change and focuses on the important issues.

This comes back to picking your battles and choosing what is worth the fight and the effort. The last thing you want is to look back on a situation and realize effort could have been redirected because of the resultant defeat. It gets better with time and experience; just keep your head up and give your best. That is all that can be asked of you. If you ever feel you or someone else is falling short, the question to always ask is: Did you give it your best? Then you can move forward and determine the next steps.

Keeping joy in the workplace and practicing meaningful recognition are key to your training to survive. These have been proven to prevent the long-term effects of burnout and compassion fatigue in the ICU. While it is best when these principles are active from the top down, it is possible to be effective as a team in recognizing and celebrating one another, creating a joyful and tolerable environment. Many ICU settings are challenging just because of the patient acuity and rhythm of the unit. When teamed with negativity and stress from leadership and other factors, maintaining joy is challenging but not impossible to accomplish.

You can be the difference by bringing joy and shining your light to make the environment a better place to work. Can we change all the factors involved? No, but we can take a look at what *can* be controlled and what *we* can do to bring joy and focus on that. This can include celebrating accomplishments—even when they are a part of the daily responsibilities. Just letting someone know they are doing a great job can be the difference between wanting to stay or go to another unit. That simple encouragement goes a long way in reminding each other you are appreciated. Paying it forward in sharing your gratitude lays the groundwork for continued joy and meaningful recognition.

You have sown the seed that will germinate and grow into something worth working toward. You may not see an immediate shift, but there will always be someone who benefits from your positive light, and that makes it worth the effort. Additionally, you will be blessed because of your willingness to appreciate others. In units where there is no lack of positivity, it is still crucial to practice this tactic in maintaining a healthy work environment. We are all human, and no one is perfect. There is always an opportunity for improvement and growth, with each one of us taking part in each other's journey. Joy trains you to survive in any ICU environment because it sets you up to thrive in the long haul.

What are the methods currently used in your facility for keeping joy in the workplace and celebrating each other? If none exist at this time, what creative ideas would you consider helpful in this area? It may be worth presenting your ideas to your manager as they come through your experience. You may be surprised by how the smallest of measures can have the biggest impact.

7

We Win When We Take Care of Ourselves

Taking care of ourselves begins with taking a self-assessment. Please refer to the self-assessment survey included to evaluate where you are now and your progress as you grow in the ICU setting. In addition to the self-assessment, the following series of questions will assist you with further understanding of how to measure your progress and growth.

How do you measure success in life and as a nurse? How do you view a successful shift?

Identifying personal views of success is a necessary step in accomplishing your set goals and continuing to grow. There are multiple right answers to these questions, but one thing that hangs up many individuals is allowing others' opinions to cloud their judgement or sway their view of success. Especially when beginning in a new environment, it could be easy to get caught up in others' frustrations and take them on as a standard to measure up to. I would also add that the negative attitude of many physicians is a frequent contributing factor and does not necessarily help the situation.

To some degree, their view is influenced by a medical model of practice that is straightforward and without room for error. Other contributors are from other nurses and fellow team members who simply do not see the full picture, are one-sided, or are just having a bad day. Even if their personality and outlook are negative and condescending, it does not define who you are nor the level of your success. The reality is that you will encounter such individuals, but do not give into the temptation to accept defeat because of someone else's unkindness.

Measure yourself up to what is right and appropriate with common sense, not based on what is pleasing to others. Did you do your best for your patients? Did you stay hydrated and nourished? Did you complete the necessary tasks for your patients? These are items that should measure success. Your definition may change over time, but the important takeaway is that you identify your goals and align your priorities with what truly matters. There is a balance between what the patient needs, what you need, the team needs, and so forth, and it is possible to find it.

How do you respond to disappointment, correction, or flak from others?

It is not possible to please everyone all of the time. Undoubtedly, someone will be upset with something we say and/or do at some point. In the same vein, there are instances where correction is warranted and may come in seemingly uncomfortable and inconvenient moments. In either case, our response in these moments determines our growth or defeat. It is better to respond with respect than feed into the anxiety of the situation, especially when we feel defensive or offended. What was your *initial* response? It is important to take an internal look in this regard to determine if changes need to be made.

If called out on something, was it legitimate?

Often when approached with a possible or real mistake, it is the natural response to be defensive or feel attacked, especially when new to a routine or process. This question is important in self-assessment because even if the calling out is not warranted, it is a good idea to take a moment and evaluate the situation. You may be able to recognize the legitimacy right away, but I offer this caution to hopefully prevent animosity and doubt in yourself. Identifying mistakes honestly and humbly helps us grow. In the same vein, recognizing when someone's approach to correct has been misguided is also important as long as you respond in confidence and not in attempts to prove them wrong or a quick judgement.

In my experience, physicians during patient rounds would occasionally bring up something that was missed overnight or even during the current shift in front of the team in a condescending way, creating an embarrassing moment. Additionally, they would correct something said in error right away. It had been easy for me in those moments to feel inferior; however, I have learned that it is better to acknowledge the issue for what it was.

If I had done something wrong, I learned from it. If they were incorrect in some way, I knew enough to respect their position and professionally share the correct information. Other instances may occur during the handoff report or during the shift from leaders. Regardless of the situation, be confident in where you are even when you know you have a way to go yet. It is better to be honest with yourself and others if there is something that you do not know, so the patient is safe.

How do you deal with stress?

Stress relief is a must in life. Add on the stress of working in the ICU and the need greatly increases. Take a moment to think of what you do outside of work to cope with stress, and remind yourself to continue those practices. You may like to read, exercise, meditate, go shopping; the list continues. Dealing with stress at work may also include taking a quick walk away from the situation or simply doing breathing exercises. Many times, you may not be able to leave the unit, *but* taking a moment to breathe in for four seconds, hold your breath for four seconds, exhale for four seconds, and repeat once or twice can make the difference.

Another aspect of taking care of ourselves is finding support by making time for ourselves and learning from the experience of others. The gift of time can be very healing for us and is a crucial step in winning. You most likely have a full plate outside of work, and the workload is also busy, making it that much more important to carve out the time to pamper yourself and truly take a break from the chaos. In doing so, you clear your head from the stress, focus on the important things in life, and can approach the work environment with a fresh perspective. Time is very precious and can get away from us very quickly.

Taking advantage of moments to reflect, heal, and replenish makes the most of what we are given and allows us to give our best in every situation. That being said, you also win when you keep yourself from overworking and take those moments to breathe. As mentioned before, use your paid time off and space your workdays enough to allow yourself to recoil. Think about the cardiac cycle in CPR. We time the compressions out just right to give the chest time to recoil and perfuse the system. The same is true for our lives. We need time in between the chaos to perfuse our system with good life and breath that feeds our souls. Let your life be influenced by what encourages you, supports you, and lifts you up.

As you hold conversations, speak words of encouragement, even about yourself. Often times, we speak negatively about ourselves without even thinking about it. I have caught myself many times over the years just reaffirming my areas of weakness rather than sharing the good things that I have accomplished and grown into. As we set goals to continue improving, we can see there is a chance to live a quality life. Think of it this way: *you* are worth it. Your life is worth it to someone else who benefits from your experience. There are many factors that could cause us to not like our jobs, but practicing these tactics reminds us of what we *do* love as ICU nurses. We need to take care of ourselves to truly take care of others.

Gleaning from the experience of those around us is a part of the journey of growing as ICU nurses. You will find one or more nurses you can confide in who have been where you are. They have made mistakes and even been very successful in their field or maybe just with life things. Leaning on their support will help you with the process of growth, cope with the stress, and continue on your journey. Having someone to share with who has been through the same battles can be very therapeutic because you do not have to explain the situation in as much detail.

You may even find someone removed from the medical field who could offer a different perspective that you may need for a situation.

It is also helpful to not discount the expertise of those with less or similar experience to yourself, as their perspective could shine a light on something you just needed to see differently. Finding common ground with your teammates can be enough to support one another and develop strong relationships with good influence. Keeping appropriate boundaries in mind, do not be afraid to share your struggles when you need support. I would only caution you to trust your instincts and know whether they are someone who you can safely open yourself up to personally with.

8

Prepping Your Go Bag

Things to Take with You Wherever You Go

As with any military strategic assignment and some wilderness situations, a go bag is a required item that equips the user for whatever may be involved in their journey. While the ingredients may differ, the ICU nurse needs a go bag as well that will travel to every assignment and location they will go to. Here is a list of what you will need to get you started:

Item 1: Trust the process.
Most things will come with time and repetition. You will have moments when you feel inadequate

and/or you will forget things, but know that you have what it takes to succeed and will become more confident as you go through each step. Remember, Rome was not built in one day! You will get there. Life is a continual, beautiful process of discovery. Just keep moving.

Item 2: Trust your gut!

If something does not feel right, bring it up to your preceptor, charge nurse, or further up the chain if needed. Instinct is something that we should not take for granted, and it grows with experience. Use your resources and do not be afraid to speak up for your patients.

Item 3: Trust your preceptor.

They have the experience to help you. Discuss the rationale and talk through the process with them. Eventually, this will apply to your charge nurses and seasoned nurses as well.

Item 4: Always ask questions!

Keep yourself open to inquiry and discovery. We are always in the process of learning, and we do not know everything. We can only limit ourselves to our full potential when we think we have nothing else to learn.

Item 5: Converse with the physicians.

Physicians are humans too! Not every physician is necessarily as approachable as you; however, that should not limit you from asking questions, provoking conversations, and clarifying details in a patient case. Often by being clear, firm, and to the point about what the patient needs will open the door to an approachable relationship. Ultimately, you are the patient's advocate, and you have the expertise to take care of them. Be open, honest, and persistent if needed so the patient gets what they need. In some ways, this builds your confidence and makes you a stronger nurse.

Item 6: Remember why you are a nurse.

You have answered the call. How you entered the nursing field may or may not be a glamorous or heart-wrenching story. It may have been just for the steady pay. Somewhere in there, however, you have the desire and passion to care for people. Keep that passion and drive alive, so when those discouraging moments come, you are reminded of the heart of the work.

Item 7: Remember what brought you to critical care.

Keeping yourself motivated is fueled by remembering what brought you here. You can see how far you have come later on, and reflect upon those pieces that have meant the most.

Item 8: Do not forget compassion and the person you are caring for.

We so easily get entangled and caught up in the busyness and tasks to accomplish that it has the tendency to distract us from the humanness of our patients. There are so many standards to follow, so much knowledge to impart, and so many items to complete in a shift. It is more impactful when others know how much we care rather than how much we know.

Item 9: The flow comes with time.

You will get better at time management; just keep working on it. Customize your time so you do not get overwhelmed with the tasks. Use a checklist if you need to, or at least have a way to track what is needed for your shift to keep yourself organized.

Item 10: Keep your goals in mind.

Set your measurable and attainable goals in place, both short-term and long-term. This will include accomplishments you pursued during your time in ICU and may include advancing your degree. Keeping them in mind motivates you to press on and give your best in your care and all that you do. Your goals may change as time goes on and life changes, but as long as you are looking forward, it makes the current situation tolerable.

Final Salutations

It is now up to you! These survival tactics will prepare you for any ICU setting and help you on your journey. While this is not an exhaustive list, these skills are enough to equip you for the challenges you will face because they can be applied however you need them. Though many of them seem like reminders of common sense, it also seems like common sense is taken for granted these days. This is especially true when encountering stressful and intense situations while still understanding the rhythm of the ICU setting. Bedside nursing continues to become more and more challenging as patient acuity and disparities become more complex, demands increase, science advances, and so on. This really is the hardest job you will ever love. The appreciation is not always verbalized. There is little praise. But the reward is great.

The job is exhausting, but is worth the effort to see lives healed, hope restored, people die with dignity, and fellow teammates supported. You can be the difference in someone else's life for the better. I know because I remember the ones who have influenced my life when I may have been "the only one." I have experienced seeing lives improve because of one person's influence. So take these skills and be the person you are made to be! You are so much more than a nurse and deserve to live a quality life. Your experience in the ICU should be rewarding and enriching, and it is up to you to make it so. It truly is all about perspective. Go with the confidence that you *are* important to the team, to your patients, to the nursing field, and to the world in which we live. You have what it takes to succeed. You will not only survive, but *thrive* in the ICU!

Self-Assessment

Use this tool in the process of orientation
and throughout your experience as a
means to keep tabs on your progress and
if there are areas in need of attention.

	Always	Often	Neutral	Sometimes	Never
I feel as though I am an important and valued member of the team.					
It is challenging for me to find my place on the team.					
I find myself overwhelmed during my shift.					
I find it difficult to ask for help.					

I feel I can manage the shift well and ask for help when needed.					
I have positive, open communication with fellow nurses to resolve conflict.					
I am concerned there is disrespect and gossip among team members that hinders patient care and teamwork.					
I feel well supported by the nurses I work with					
I feel I give an adequate handoff report and ask appropriate questions when receiving the report.					
I feel I can continue to learn and grow in this environment as a nurse.					

How Do I Survive This?

This may be a question you ask yourself or hear others ask in the critical care setting and experience. For any critical care nurse, in any setting and with any level of experience, the challenges that they face present themselves in similar ways. As nurses in today's healthcare setting, we need support with accessible and usable tools to be the caregivers and providers we know we can be. Let this tool kit be the start of blooming where you are planted and exploring the adventure that comes with finding joy in the journey. There are many tools available that I hope you will be encouraged to find following this read.

We all have something to give in the area we are in. The unprecedented times we live in have introduced challenges we did not know we could overcome, while pushing many nurses to the limit. In whatever capacity you serve as a critical care nurse and wherever your experience takes you, remember you were made for this and your contributions do not go unnoticed. We cannot fix every part of the broken system, but we can and will make the difference we have been created to make as we choose to do our best, give our best, and be our best.

About the Author

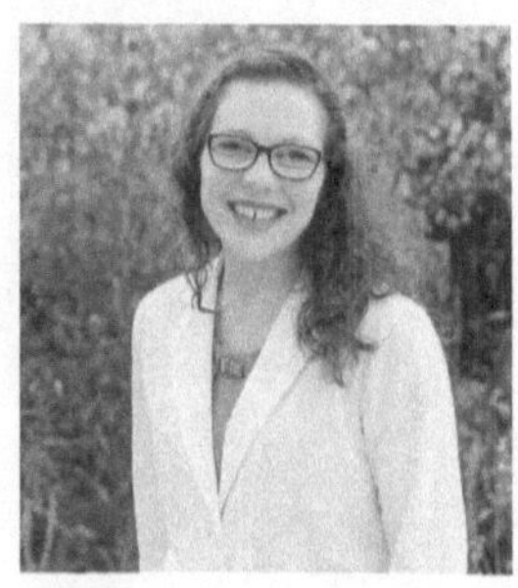

Rachel Larcom is a registered nurse and family nurse practitioner with over a decade's experience in cardiac care, specifically over six years in the open-heart CVICU environment. From the early years on, she has had a passion for imparting knowledge to and educating nurses to help them feel empowered in their field. She also serves as a copastor with her husband, Robert, at Rock Church of Lancaster County, located in Quarryville, Pennsylvania, where they live.